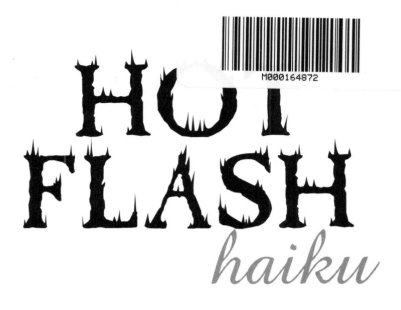

HOT FLASH

haiku

JENNIFER BASYE SANDER AND PAULA MUNIER

Aadamsmedia

AVON, MASSACHUSETTS

Published by
Adams Media, a division of F+W Media, Inc.
57 Littlefield Street, Avon, MA 02322. U.S.A.
www.adamsmedia.com

ISBN-10: 1-60550-364-9
ISBN-13: 978-1-60550-364-6

Printed in the United States of America.

10 9 8 7 6 5 4 3 2 1

Library of Congress Cataloging-in-Publication Data
is available from publisher.

This publication is designed to provide accurate and authoritative information with regard to the subject matter covered. It is sold with the understanding that the publisher is not engaged in rendering legal, accounting, or other professional advice. If legal advice or other expert assistance is required, the services of a competent professional person should be sought.

—From a Declaration of Principles jointly adopted by a Committee of the American Bar Association and a Committee of Publishers and Associations

Many of the designations used by manufacturers and sellers to distinguish their product are claimed as trademarks. Where those designations appear in this book and Adams Media was aware of a trademark claim, the designations have been printed with initial capital letters.

This book is available at quantity discounts for bulk purchases.
For information, please call 1-800-289-0963.

DEDICATION

For Carol and Renee, who from the age of fifteen have
shared my every hormonal challenge . . . we're still hot!
And a special thanks to our mothers, who never told us
it would be like this.

ACKNOWLEDGMENTS

We'd like to thank each other, and many of the talented women who've attended Jennifer's "Write by the Lake" writer's retreats (*www.writebythelake.com*) and contributed their own haikus to this project: Sherry Crum, Maridel Bowes, Dawn Larimore, Catherine Crusade, Laura Lynne Powell, and Virginia Weigand. We'd also like to thank all of the folks at Adams Media, notably: Karen Cooper, who always believed in this project; Wendy Simard, who helped count and rearrange syllables as well as edit the book; and Michelle Kelly, who created such a fun design for the book. A special thanks to Casey Ebert, Frank Rivera, Phil Sexton, Leslie Hendrickson, Sue Beale, Matt Glazer, Jon Ackerman, Matt LeBlanc, Beth Gissinger, Maureen D'Haene, Meredith O'Hayre, and Laura Daly.

Contents

Introduction

But you have to go through a lot of hormones first. It all starts when you get your first period, and doesn't let up until you finally get rid of it, several decades and PMS, pregnancy, lactation, and perimenopause later. Then you hit menopause—and the real fun starts.

Life as you know it is over—and life as you never dreamed it begins. But between that initial flush—*is it hot in here or is it just me?*—and the last hot hormonal hurrah lies a country in which you must explore all the peaks and valleys of the feminine principle. Denial, anger, bargaining, depression—you'll wallow in them all before you come to accept the new, improved, post-menopausal you. Yes, you may grieve for your old pre-menopausal self, but do it with wit and wisdom and before you can say, "Pass the wild yam cream," you'll find that you have become the woman you were destined to become.

We're all works in progress—but Oh! What progress! Look at us! We're not little girls any more, and we're not little old ladies . . . yet.

We're grown women now
No hot flash in the pan, just
Hot, hotter, hottest!

CHAPTER 1

denial

"*As a graduate of the Zsa Zsa Gabor*

School of Creative Mathematics, I honestly

do not know how old I am."

—ERMA BOMBECK

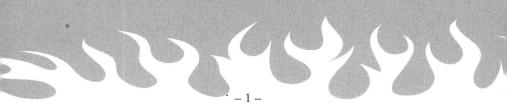

My upper lip feels

Moist and warmer than my face.

Is this the first sign?

Dry is good for wit

And clothes and babies and air

But oh God, not *there*.

Another wrinkle.

When did you arrive? *Today?*

You're **not** welcome here.

What fresh hormone hell
Is this? Happy, sad, horny

All in a minute.

What to do with next Fifty years of my one and

Only life? Play hard!

Black coffee fuels my

Pondering of future lives

Let *caffeine dreams* rule!

Credit card. Shoe sale.

Dangerous combination.

Willpower. Fades. Fast.

How old am I? I

Used to know but now it's gone.

Drew a blank again.

My mom wore girdles
That left welts and now we're bound
In Spanx. That's progress?

Seaweed wrap: Did I
Mix up the spa brochure with
The sushi menu?

I *swore* I'd never

Wear sensible shoes ever

But look at me now.

I *swore* I'd never

Answer to the name Grandma

But look at me now.

I *swore* I'd never

Fall in love (or lust) again

But look at me now.

I wrap my hands, pull
On my red boxing gloves and
Throw the first punch. Hard.

If I could turn back

Time, I'd look just like *Cher* did

Before surgery.

This cannot be me—
The *wrinkled* mug I see now
I don't recognize.

Forgetfulness: On
The stair landing, was it *up*

Or *down* I'm going?

Erotic ideas

Float up from nowhere. It seems

Sex is on my mind.

Fifty is the new

Forty...Sixty is the new

Fifty...I've lost count.

We still share so much:

Remember when we were kids?

(Yeah, I don't either.)

Gossip with my friends,

A good book to read at night.

This is what I need.

My MUSCLES ache though
My smile still works like a charm
(BUT OTHER PARTS DON'T.)

Domestic goddess?

Not. Last touched the oven in 1998.

When did men our age
Get so stuffy and boring?

Let's date younger men.

Say it loud, say it
Proud: I am a grandmother!
Oh my f—ing god.

My sons say that I'm
Not old, I am beautiful.
I raised those boys right.

My daughter says that

I'm beautiful, too, but then

She looks just like me.

When I saunter by

Men still do a doubletake.

They think I'm a babe.

Never felt so young!

I swear! I'm not growing old!

(Hello, denial.)

There are some young men
Who bait me with their **bold** stares

Careful what you want.

Other women cry
Over new wrinkles but I
JUST SAY "WHAT THE F—K."

The mirror sees me
Now, but I see the same girl
I saw at sixteen.

Stuck in the middle
Of my life, waiting for…what?

TIME TO GET MOVING.

Slip on a little

BLACK dress and go out *dancing*

WHILE YOU STILL CAN TWIRL.

When did pantyhose
Become the enemy? Let
Those old gams go bare.

My mom is shrinking
For the first time in my life
I'm as tall as she.

My *baby girl* is
Having a *baby girl*. How
Is this possible?

WHERE IS MY CHECKBOOK?

With my keys, my bag, my comb
Somewhere in the house....

I still have my hair

And my teeth but where on earth
Did my eyebrows go?

There's a man my age

With all his hair. Quick! Lure him

In for a test drive.

Older men smile at
    Me but I'm not old enough

            To date my dad. **Yet.**

CHAPTER 2

anger

"It is utterly false and cruelly arbitrary

to put all the play and learning into

childhood, all the work into middle age,

and all the regrets into old age."

—MARGARET MEAD

"AGE APPROPRIATE"

Is just another way to

Keep this old broad down.

All the sit-ups and

Diets in the world won't beat

THAT SLY MENOPOT.

If **EX-HUSBANDS** were
Like **FED-EX**, I could send him

To an obscure spot.

A cruel magic act:

GRAVITY TUGS, I GO FROM

Woman to Shar Pei.

I DON'T LIKE my knees
Once so STRONG and FLEXIBLE
Now so SORE and WEAK.

Where did my looks go?

Over to that young girl there?

I want them back now.

If I use this cream

My pores will shrink, my lips swell,
And pigs will soon fly.

Burn your bras, corsets, Girdles, pantyhose, and Spanx!

Let freedom wriggle!

Whenever someone
My age gets her face lifted

IT PISSES ME OFF.

I pluck, tweeze, shave, wax.

Worse than dealing with crabgrass.

Argh—always grows back.

OLD LADY HAIR on
My chin. When did I begin
To look LIKE MY DOG?

Who says I must lose
My *f—k-me* pumps? (WELL, BESIDES
MY PODIATRIST....)

Old boyfriends

look oh

So old now, but still I **lust**

For the one I **lost.**

What about *my* needs?
So long ignored for others
But starting to show....

Hungry ALL the time

CRAVING CAKE, but what am I

Really HUNGRY for?

E-mail, IM, text

Messages—JUST TELL ME that

You love me OUT LOUD.

All this talk about
Cougars…we've all been growling
And prowling since birth!

What is the point of
Shaving my legs when I know
He can't get it up?

My youngest child is

Nearly grown and now it's time
To get a life. SHIT.

Fooled for the last time!

Heard twenty years of *sweet talk*
And just now caught on.

Three balls to juggle,

Work, kids, and oops! Just dropped the Husband ball. Again.

Will he call, why won't
He call, should I call him? I'm
Too old for this shit!

It's so easy to

WORK AND WORK AND WORK AND WORK

Why can't I *play* hard?

THEY SAY THAT THE FACE

YOU HAVE AT FIFTY IS THE

FACE YOU DESERVE. RIGHT.

Boxing builds **STRONG** bones,

My young trainer tells me, **SO**

Watch me **POUND** that bag.

Every woman I Know says she needs **more sex**. So,

Guys, what's up with that?

To those products that

Promise to *lift* this, tuck that

I say: *Whatever.*

We women of a
Certain age are told to age
"*Gracefully.*" No way!

What to wear over
40—no short skirts, no bare
Midriffs, nothing fun.

In *Mexico* they

Say "**La Meno.**" Sounds nice but

It's an insult…*not!*

Wrinkles, **hot flashes,** **Night sweats.** I don't think we're in Kansas any more.

CHAPTER 3

bargaining

"*It's sad to grow old, but nice to ripen.*"

—Brigitte Bardot

BOTOX OR BANGS, that

Is the question I ponder.

I choose BANGS—for now.

*M*y real breasts might sag.

Time to think about a *lift*?

Haul them up *higher*?

The best things in life

Are free, but only if you

Price yourself high 'nuf.

Where is Mr. Right?

Still single at forty-four,

Found Mr. Right Now.

Don't fence me in, BUT
Little retaining walls here
And there couldn't hurt.

My lover left me.

Too late to take another?

Ah, younger brother!

FROWNING will straighten
Out all of your *laugh lines*—are
They really that bad?

The best thing about
Long, hot bubble baths is that
The wrinkles don't last.

Red wine is the best

Cures what ails you, and then some—

All women need it.

My toes need some love

A delicious pedicure.

I can afford it.

Knee brace works just fine
Attitude also helps to
Keep me standing tall.

He looked like Brad Pitt

Or Brad Pitt's older brother....

Either way, he's mine.

I'm always tired.
So I lie awake for hours
Thinking up new tricks.

Focus on my waist

So small and tight and well-toned.

Don't look at my neck!

I'd trade my laugh lines

For his little love handles

Any time. DAMN MEN.

On bad days I feel

One hundred and one years old

On good days I don't.

Give me a man who
Thinks a grandma is *sexy*,
And I'll give you mine.

I WILL GROW OLDER

On MY OWN terms, MY OWN rules,

THE WAY I WANT TO!

House under water,

Stocks worth zip, savings all gone.

WHAT RETIREMENT?

Ooooo, he looks so good.
Not my husband, not my man.

But still, I can dream….

I eye the handbag.

Looking at the price I think,
Will this give me peace?

He is going gray,

He is going bald, but is
He going my way?

Love IS BETTER THE
SECOND TIME AROUND, AND THE

THIRD, AND THE FOURTH, AND....

SECOND CHANCES ARE
OVERRATED. So let's try
For *third time's a charm.*

"You're not my mother

Yet," says my own mom to me.

A BAD DAY COMING.

Dad says never let

The **bastards** get you down so

SLEEP ALONE—for now.

Silk pajamas and *Satin sheets*—all dressed up for

Sexy Solitaire.

I know they say that

You will lose your libido

Ha! I DON'T THINK SO.

It happened one night
A clever explorer found

My lost vagina.

So if this be the
Winter of my life, then I'll

Simply pray for snow.

One last teenager
To get through the worst years and
Then we can both *fly*.

MEN are like trains, if
You don't catch this one then just
Catch the next damn train.

If I'm supposed to

Dry up like an old prune then

Why am I so wet?

Chocolate is fine but

There's only one way to scratch

My itch for candy.

I used to buy shoes

But now when I am stressed out,
I breathe. Namaste.

Took a whole day off

Just for me. *Beach, massage, chick*

Flick. And home again.

There's a middle-aged
Woman poised at the surf's edge

"Dive in," I whisper.

If men think about

SEX every seven seconds,

WHY CAN'T WE GET LAID?

No more periods

Means no more worries, so drop
Those pants now, Mister.

He's 26 and

Back home with Mom. Now it's time
To teach him to fish.

He was 15 years
Younger and I balked but now
I do know better.

Yoga, massage, all
That body work makes me think
Think I'm **HOT**. Again.

I let him in and

I know it's not forever...

When is it ever?

Mr. Right Now had

A heart attack and now I

See that I love him.

CHAPTER 4

depression

"The really frightening thing about middle age is that you know you'll grow out of it."

—DORIS DAY

Once I was *so* hot

But now hotter than ever

Many times a day.

How many times can
You *break your poor heart* and then
Will it whole again?

Got no clue about

What my teens are doing now

ARE THEY GROWN UP YET?

I think of old loves...

What might have happened with him

Instead of this life?

I have three chances

For a broken heart. Count them:

TWO SONS, ONE HUSBAND.

My daughter is so *Beautiful*, just like I was

Thirty years ago.

The print is so small
I can't see to read without
Bringing it up close.

Bad news on TV:
I heard last night that it's your
Hands that show your age.

Creases like canyons…

My own harsh geography…

Laugh lines make me blue.

Dining alone now.

Break out a nice pinot and

Drink to solitude.

"My **thickening** waist"

Sounds sickening, but yet it

Will soon be mine too.

Old boyfriend stopped by

I was surprised by his hair—

Once so long, now gone.

My boss is younger
My physician is YOUNGER
My man is younger.

Nordstrom's or Walmart

Good credit or bad—that's your

Retail therapy.

Note to self: NO MORE

CRYiNG, EaTiNG, FEELiNG SaD.

LEaVE PiTY BEHiND.

No more making those
New Year's Resolutions to
Get laid. **I GIVE UP.**

One *martini* for

Me, one *martini* for you

Girls' night out, again.

Since when do men like
To talk about their feelings?
Since they hit 50.

The sex is great but
Then I just wish he'd go home.

(I've become a man.)

I used to sing my

Babies to sleep. Now I sing

My Self Electric.

That used to be me
On the beach with the kids, now

It's just me and sea.

All those obnoxious

Teenagers grown and gone, now
I miss their bad selves.

FINALLY there's time

For me. What the hell will I

Ever do with it?

Alone in my bed

Sprawled across the sheets solo

Too much empty space.

Work, kids, two husbands
All those crowded years, who knew

I'd be lonely now?

There are days when life
Seems so *beautiful* that all
I can do is cry.

There are days when life

Seems so terrible that all

I CAN DO IS LAUGH.

CHAPTER 5

acceptance

"We turn not older with years,

but newer every day."

—EMILY DICKINSON

Old, older, oldest
Young, younger, youngest. In truth,
Who's to say who's whom?

He's *cute*, he's *sexy*

You think he's too young for you.

THINK AGAIN, GIRLFRIEND.

I'm wrinkled, so what.

I'm menopausal, so what.

I'm still here, so *there*.

ME? INVISIBLE?

MAYBE TO YOUNG BEEFCAKE, BUT

NOT TO YOUNG GRANDKIDS!

I rage, resist, grieve.

Body thickens, sweats, transforms.

But wisdom soothes me.

My old dog can't move

Very fast and needs to pee

All the time. **Ditto!**

He's **hot**, and half your

Age, so skinny-dip with him

That's **naughty** and nice!

"Freedom to focus,"

Jamie Lee Curtis suggests,

Arrives at fifty.

*B*ad news for you—they
Say I get the same effect
By eating *chocolate.*

EASY DECISIONS:

Head for Häagen-Dazs, bypass

The swimsuit section.

Now I understand:

My mother never told me

Because she forgot.

A small *nightly thrill*

When the dinner part is done

And the night begun.

Lost reading glasses?

I need them for many tasks....
Like finding glasses.

Martinis are the

Best medicine to relax

And let my cares go.

Magazines tell me
The next few years will be rough

So I don't read them.

High school reunions

Don't scare me. Forget prom queens.
I'm the rich bitch now.

Big hair, *big* jewelry

My fashion statements increase

Look at me now, world!

Now who would have guessed

Years ago, I would ever

Think bald was sexy?

Nothing is too hard
I am unstoppable now—
Able to achieve.

AT NIGHT THE WIND HOWLS
I AM SAFE UNDER MY QUILT
SURE OF MY OLD HOUSE.

At the mountaintop
Legs sore, but spirit is pleased
I could climb so high.

A small feather says

"With your children grown and gone,

It's your turn to soar."

The house is now clean

I enjoy it by myself.

Sit quietly now.

On the clearance rack

Of life, I'm one good bargain

Can you afford me?

I touch myself there.

Yes, it still works quite nicely.

My best working part.

Sexy skirt feels good
Swishes when I walk down steps
Toward my rendezvous.

I still wear high heels

Yes, the higher the better

To show off, that is.

I still wear high heels

Short skirts and plunging necklines

'Cause I'm not dead yet.

My old man, he is

Shrinking in more ways than one.

Still he's *my* old man.

Hard work to climb high.

Best to try it with your friends,

Reach the peak in groups.

Aging gracefully

Is for suckers. I prefer

Raging gracefully.

The older I get
The more I fall in love with
My own damn sweet self.

WHAT THIS HAIKU AND

I HAVE IN COMMON: NEITHER

HAS A PERIOD

Marriage, kids, divorce,

Empty nest. Everyone flown

But me. Time to soar!

Yoga winds me up

Twists me around and then it

Allows me to sleep.

Short hair is best, or

So they say. I let mine grow

Long and I love it.

A warm bath, silk sheets,

Candlelight, and solitude:

SATISFACTION NOW.

My mother, me, my

Daughter, my granddaughter, we

ARE A LEGACY.

Sophia Loren's

Mom says she's still horny at 80. That's good genes.

Always slept so late,
But now I wake up early.
The sunrise moves me.

Just when you think that

Your baby days are over,

The grandchild arrives!

He may be gray and

Paunchy and slightly stooped but

Still he's **hot** to me.

I may be lined—*not!*
And a little lumpy but
Still he's hot for me.

Two marriages, three Kids, one grandchild…now that's what I call dividends.

Three high school girls met

Thirty-five years ago and

We're still giggling now.

Full moon shines on my

Little cottage on the lake

Peace in my own time.

Long walk through the bogs
With the dogs on a cool spring
Morning clears my head.

Thighs that wiggle and
Glutes that jiggle but still I
Wriggle into you.

My middle child, the

One who made me so crazy

Still calls me "Mommy."

Chocolate or sex? What

Kind of silly choice is that?

Indulge in both. Now.

He's got all his hair,

And a six-pack to die for,

And he's my age. **SCORE!**

Men over 50

May need Viagra to get

It up. So drug him.

The day I let Doc

McKnife "lift" my face is the

Day I move to France.

There are few words more
Beautiful in any tongue

Than *Portofino*.

When the going gets

Tough, the tough grab a glass of

Red wine and chocolate.

Recite the *Aging Gracefully Rules* and then throw Them out the window.

16,000 WORDS

A day is a lot of talk

Bask in the silence.

Younger men don't mind
If you make **more** money or
Like to be on top.

Just when you think that

You're so over all that jazz,

Along comes a horn.

When love comes so late

In life there's nothing to do

But get on with it.

In Paris they say
The best French beauty secret
Is this: *Self-esteem.*

I feel in my bones

That life is just beginning

Once again, loudly.

ABOUT THE AUTHORS

Jennifer Basye Sander has been creating successful book products since 1983, when she published her first book, *The Sacramento Women's Yellow Pages*. She is also the author, coauthor, or ghostwriter of more than thirty books, including the recent gift book hits *Wear More Cashmere* and *The Martini Diet*. Several times a year, she leads women's writing retreat weekends in South Lake Tahoe, "Write by the Lake." Jennifer lives in Granite Bay, California.

Paula Munier is an acquisitions editor by day and writer by night, the author of *Yes, We Can!: 365 Ways to Make America a Better Place*; *On Being Blonde*; the young adult novel *Emerald's Desire*; and coauthor of *101 Things You (and John McCain) Didn't Know about Sarah Palin*. As the Director of Acquisitions and Innovation for Adams Media, she also acquires and develops nonfiction series and stand-alone titles for the trade market. When she's not hot flashing, she works up a good sweat boxing. Paula lives in Boston, Massachusetts.